CBD HEMP OIL

Everything You Need to Know About CBD Hemp Oil

Table of Contents

Introduction 1

Chapter 1: Getting to Know Hemp 5

Chapter 2: Hemp versus Marijuana 19

Chapter 3: Benefits and Side Effects of CBD 23

Chapter 4: How CBD works in the body 37

Chapter 5: CBD Hemp Oil 49

Chapter 6: Different Types of CBD Hemp Oil.........61

Chapter 7: How to Use CBD Hemp Oil.......................73

Chapter 8: Guide for Buying CBD Hemp Oil...........79

Chapter 9: Is CBD Hemp Oil Good for Pets? 85

Conclusion 95

Thank you!..97

INTRODUCTION

History shows that one of the first plants utilized as usable fiber was the industrial hemp or hemp. This versatile, durable and naturally-soft fiber plant was refined into clothing, paper, textiles, oil, food, biofuel, medicine, rope, animal feeds, insulation, paint and biodegradable plastics.

But did you know that, hemp was also used as money or legal tender in America for more than 200 years? People during those times could pay taxes with hemp. It was so valuable in England and America that when farmers failed to grow cannabis in their fields, they were sent to jail or penalized.

Sadly, the golden years of hemp eventually ended. Many nations, such as the United States of America, regulated the production and use of hemp. In 1937, the cultivation and commercial sale of cannabis varieties was strictly monitored by virtue of

Marijuana Tax Act. Forty-seven years after, all types of cannabis were classified as a Schedule I drug under Controlled Substances Act of 1970. Since hemp was part of this plant species, growing it inside United States became a taboo.

For many years, lawmakers and farmers fought to decriminalize the cultivation of hemp in the U.S. Finally, hope became apparent when the US Farm Bill of 2014 allowed different states that passed their industrial hemp legislation to cultivate the plant for research and development purposes. These states included the following: Colorado, Oregon and Kentucky, all three of which were already conducting pilot projects of growing hemp. Many states followed and soon enough, American farmers were reacquainting themselves with hemp's industrial benefits after a very long period of strict prohibition.

The possible repeal of prohibition and regulation resulted to the passage of The Industrial Hemp Farming Act of 2015. If it passed into law, this will end the federal restrictions to grow industrial hemp in U.S., and remove it under Schedule I classification of controlled substance. To date, hemp under this classification is considered a dangerous drug, no different from ecstasy, heroin and LSD.

CHAPTER 1

GETTING TO KNOW HEMP

Hemp is considered as a highly-sustainable and renewable resource which can easily thrive in almost any climate and soil conditions across the world. "Industrial hemp" is referred to as plant Cannabis sativa L. with delta-9 tetrahydrocannabinol (THC) concentration of 0.3% on dry-weight basis. It is based on Section 7606 of Agricultural Appropriations Act of 2014.

Over 30 countries produce different varieties of industrial hemp. In 2011, China became the top producer and world supplier of hemp. Chile and the European Union followed closely as second and third respectively. The thriving potential of hemp market attracted Canada to produce more. In 2013, the nation managed to reach an annual crop high of 66,700 acres.

The Hemp Industries Association (HIA) has estimated an average total retail value of $620 million for clothing, building materials, food products, CBD oil and other hemp-containing products.

It was once the top major crop of U.S. but because it is deemed illegal, raw material has to be imported from other countries. United States is one of the largest importers of industrial hemp. It is not illegal for the country to import raw products of hemp inside the country. Hemp Industry Association reported that every year, U.S. importation of hemp reached about $500 million.

The Re-emergence of Hemp Industry

When CNN featured, back in in 2013, a documentary entitled "Charlotte's Web cannabis", an increased demand of CBD producing hemp spread across the US. In Kentucky, a legislation to promote hemp farming as one of major development program of the state was passed to assist tobacco farmers who are suffering from drastic absence of market for their crops. The state of Kentucky strongly lobbied to make hemp production legal and won.

As of 2017, 31 states in United States were able to legalize hemp production. This includes the states of: Colorado, California, Indiana, Montana, Maine, North Dakota, North Carolina, Oregon, South Carolina, Tennessee, Vermont and West Virginia.

Other states also passed legislations which authorized pilot studies or researches to grow industrial hemp plants. These include Utah, Nebraska, Kentucky, Illinois, Hawaii, Delaware and Connecticut.

Resolutions that support revisions of federal rules and regulations for commercial production of hemp were later adopted by the National Conference of State Legislatures and the National Association of State Departments of Agriculture.

In Utah, people who possess CBD supplements are exempted from penalties imposed under Controlled Substances Act if they have a Hemp Extract Registration Card which is signed by an authorized neurologist. The neurologist must indicate in the card that the person is showing symptoms of intractable epilepsy or is in need of the substance for health reasons. A regular submission of evaluation data to the Utah Department of Health is another task that the neurologist needs to comply. The user must also obtain a certificate of extract analysis from hemp's product seller.

In New Zealand, anyone who wants to use CBD hemp products would have to seek the approval of Health Ministry. Cannabidiol remains as a class B1 controlled drug under Misuse of Drugs Act and a prescription drug under Medicines Act. Before the changes in the rules, the sole way to get prescription was to get the Minister of Health's personal approval. At present, doctors can prescribe CBD to patients who are in dire need of its benefits.

In Canada, CBD is a Schedule II drug and is only obtainable with prescription.

In Europe, CBD is listed in both EU Cosmetics Ingredient Database and EU Novel Food Catalogue. However, crude extracts of hemp are not listed-- only synthetic CBD. A position paper for regulatory framework was issued by the European Industrial Hemp Association. At present, there are hemp varieties that are grown legally in the western part of Europe. One of them is "Fedora 17", a cannabis plant with 1% cannabidiol (CBD) and 0.1% THC.

In Sweden, CBD is not classified. One product that contains CBD and THC, called Sativex, is available upon prescription. It brings relief for illnesses such as severe spasticity, a symptom of Multiple Sclerosis.

In the United Kingdom, people with Multiple Sclerosis can avail, upon prescription, a CDB spray which is laden with delta-9-THC. On December 31, 2016, CBD products with the purpose of addressing medical conditions were classified as medicines by the Medicines and Healthcare products Regulatory Agency (MHRA). However, a regulatory approval must first be secured for medical claims before they can be commercially available for users.

In Switzerland, CBD products are legally sold in the country and not subjected to Swiss Narcotics Act. However, the product must contain less than 1% THC since THC is still illegal there.

Varieties of Hemp

Hemp has many varieties. Each of them offers unique characteristics and nutritional values to people using them. The most-sought after variety which is used to manufacture CBD hemp oil has very high concentration content.

Fiber and oilseed varieties of Cannabis are known as industrial hemp. These varieties do not contain the addictive component that is prohibited in many countries.

Different varieties of Cannabis grow at different density conditions. They are also harvested at different periods.

Industrial hemp varieties seeding rate differ per acre. The recommended seeding rate to produce hemp fiber is 60 pounds per acre (30-35 plants for every square foot). Finola is seeded at 30 pounds per acre while Crag , USO 31 and USO 14 are seeded at 20 pounds per acre

Cultivation of Cannabis Varieties across the World

The USDA used an extensive range of hemp varieties in their breeding program during the time of Lyster H. Dewey until his retirement in 1930s. They named the varieties as Simple Leaf, Michigan Early and Minnesota No. 8. Other varieties which they bred but became extinct were Chington, Ferramington, Kymington, Tochimington and Chinamington.

At present, there are many cultivars or varieties of hemp in different seed banks across the world.

The European Union (EU) certified 26 hemp varieties to be cultivated. All these varieties contain low to almost zero levels of tetrahydrocannabinol (THC). The most sought-after variety of industrial hemp produces about 1-5% of pure botanical cannabidiol (CBD) oil.

In Canada, the common varieties which are approved by Health Canada List of Approved Cultivars:

- USO 14

- Finola (formerly called FIN 314)

- Crag

- USO 31

- Alyssa

- Felina 34

These hemp varieties are part of the 2007 List of Approved Cultivars based on Organization for Economic Co-operation and Development (OECD). The OECD is an economic development organization founded in 1961 with main office in Paris, France. One of the 30 members is the United States.

The largest Cannabis collection in the world is the "germplasm" which is now preserved at N.I.Vavilov Research Institute of Plant Industry (VIR). The VIR collection before World War II numbered at about 1400 accessions but today there are only 491 remaining.

Finland's Dr. J.C. Callaway bred the oilseed cultivar Finola with VIR germplasm and became a success. Now, it is grown in various northern countries. Finola is known as the earliest maturing hemp variety and can produce a great amount of seeds. It contains optimum amounts of omega-3 and omega -6 fatty acids. Research shows that compared to other oilseed varieties, Finola has higher amount of SDA and GLA fatty acids.

2017 List of Approved Cannabis sativa L. Industrial Hemp Cultivars

The following hemp varieties are licensed for 2017 commercial cultivation pursuant to Industrial Hemp Regulations Subsection 39 (1). The list shows the countries where they are cultivated.

- Alyssa - Canada

- Anka - Canada

- Canda - Canada

- CanMa - Canada

- Carmagnola -Italy

- Carmen - Canada

- CFX-1 - Canada

- CFX-2 -Canada

- Crag - Canada

- CRS-1 -Canada

- CS - Italy

TOM WHISTLER

- Delores - Canada

- Deni - Canada

- ESTA-1 - Canada

- Fasamo - Germany

- Fedrina 74 - France

- Felina 34 - France

- Ferimon - France

- Fibranova - Italy

- Fibriko - Hungary

- Fibrimon 24 -France

- Fibrimon 56 -France

- FINOLA - Canada (Finland)

- Georgina - Canada

- GranMa - Canada

- Grandi - Canada

- Joey - Canada

- Judy - Canada

- Jutta - Canada

- Katani - Canada

- Kompolti - Hungary

- Kompolti Hibrid TC - Hungary

- Kompolti Sargaszaru - Hungary

- Lovrin 110 - Romania

- Petera - Canada

- Picolo - Canada

- Silesia - Canada

- UC-RGM - Canada

- Uniko B - Hungary

- USO 14 - Canada (Ukraine)

- USO 31 - Canada (Ukraine)

- Victoria - Canada

- X-59 (Hemp Nut) - Canada

- Yvonne - Canada

- Zolotonosha 11 - Canada (Ukraine)

- Zolotonosha 15 - Canada (Ukraine)

All the seeds used to produce industrial hemp in Canada are required to be of pedigreed status or certified based on Subsection 14 (3) of Industrial Hemp Regulations (IHR). Farmers with saved seeds must be Certified-seeds before they are allowed to be planted. They must request for inspection and need official seed tags as evidence that they comply with the regulations.

The regulation also restricts direct importation of the above-mentioned seeds if they are not recognized by Seed Certification Schemes (SCS), of which Canada is an active member. The country is also a member of two other schemes – the Association of Official Seed Certifying Agencies (AOSCA) and Organization for Economic Cooperation and Development (OECD).

Countries Producing Industrial Hemp

France is now the leading producer of hemp in the world. It produces over 70% of the total global output. The second in rank is China which provides a quarter of the world production. Other nations which contribute to the overall hemp output in the market are Europe, North Korea and Chile.

Industrial hemp are now grown and supplied by more than 30 countries across the world including Austria, Australia, Chile, Canada, China, Denmark, Egypt, Finland, Great Britain, Greece, Germany, Hungary, Italy, India, Japan, Korea, New Zealand, Netherlands, Portugal, Poland, Russia, Romania, Spain, Slovenia, Switzerland, Sweden, Turkey, Thailand and Ukraine.

Companies in United Kingdom, United States, Canada and Germany are among the many that process hemp seeds into a number of other commodities including: cosmetics, food products and textile-grade fibers. British production targets horses' beddings. Germany and United Kingdom stopped commercial production for a long time then resumed in 1990s.

Hemp was believed to be one of the earliest grown plants and is still thriving at present. In 8000 BC, archeologists discovered a site in Japan's Oki Islands that contained cannabis of the Achenes variety. But this isn't the first and only known use of the plant in ancient history.

There's plenty of evidence that even the earliest civilizations made use of the plant for many different reasons—some, not too different from how we use it today.

The beneficial uses of hemp can be dated back to Neolithic Age, where fiber imprints have been found in China's Yangshao pottery culture. Hemp was mainly utilized by the ancient Chinese to make ropes, clothes, shoes and paper. The Greek historian Herodotus, in 480 BC, wrote that Scythia inhabitants used to inhale hemp-seed smoke during their ritual rites and for recreation.

CHAPTER 2

HEMP VERSUS MARIJUANA

Both hemp and marijuana come from the Cannabis sativa L. specie. The term cannabis is oftentimes associated with the more recreational use of the plant, often smoked by people who are looking to get "high". The mislabeling of marijuana as a recreational yet dangerous drug has significant affected the marketing of industrial hemp, with many people thinking that these two things are the same.

THEY ARE NOT.

It is unfortunate that they are mistakenly regarded as similar because of their tetrahydrocannabinol (THC) content. However, the quantity of THC in hemp is only about .3 to 1.5% THC, much less when compared to the 20% THC content of marijuana.

Hemp is not marijuana, and marijuana is not hemp. They are also genetically different. Each has its distinct uses and chemical components.

Even their cultivation methods are not the same. The fruits and blooms of hemp produces strong fibers and seeds. On the other hand, Marijuana flowers and buds are often used to produce psychoactive effects.

Hemp also contains a high-amount of concentrated cannabidiol or CBD which acts as a neutralizer of psychoactive effects that its THC bring. It does not give the same psychoactive sensation that marijuana does simply because the small amount of THC in it is processed immediately by the body.

The hemp plant is can be easily grown outdoors to produce maximum yields and size. It does not require pesticides or a high-amount of water to thrive. As it grows, it can actually help with detoxifying the soil, removes any traces of carbon dioxide in the air and prevents soil erosion problem.

Marijuana on the other hand needs grow-room conditions with a sustained oxygen level, CO2, humidity, temperature and stable light in order to achieve the optimum level of THC content. It is far more delicate than hemp as well.

- Industrial hemp is categorized as agricultural crop. Marijuana and other drug variety of Cannabis plant is horticultural crop.

- Drug varieties are planted without spacing and pruning while oilseed/fiber varieties are planted like pulp wood trees.

- Drug varieties which are grown as drug crops give you drugs. Oilseed varieties grown as fiber crops give oilseed. Fiber varieties grown as fiber crops give fibers.

- When different varieties are grown with dual purpose, this basically doubles your harvest and you can maximize the benefit of the plant itself. If you grow oilseed and fiber varieties as dual purpose crop, they yield fiber and oilseed. If you grow oilseed and fiber varieties as drug crop, they would not produce drugs.

- Hemp seeding rates are measurable by pounds per acre. Drug-varieties seeds are measured by ounces per acre.

- Oilseed varieties seeding rates are about 20-30 pounds per acre. Fiber varieties are rates are 40-90 pounds per acre. Cannabis drug varieties seeding rates are at 18-48 ounces per acre.

Marijuana and other drug-type varieties of Cannabis utilizes the flowers of female plants. Males are cut down or pulled out because they do not yield the same effects.

Industrial hemp varieties grow up to about 16 feet high. They have strong, long stalks with very few branches. They can be bred to produce maximum amount of seed and fiber. They are grown in 100-300 plants per square yard high densities.

Some varieties are typically shorter, bred to produce maximum branching, and not allowed to seed. They are grown densely to yield more drug-producing leaves and flowers.

CHAPTER 3

BENEFITS AND SIDE EFFECTS OF CBD

CBD or cannabidiol is the main component found in the industrial hemp variety of cannabis. It has a molecular mass of about 314.4636 with formula $C_{21}H_{30}O_2$.

It is one of 113 active cannabis cannabinoids, and is considered a major phytocannabinoid which accounts to about 40% of hemp-extracted components. It does not give the same intoxicating effect of marijuana, but provides anti-psychotic and anti-stress benefits.

Various research and studies done throughout the decades show that cannabinoids or CBD actively interact with the endogenous cannabinoid system (ECS) of the body. This particular body system is complex, but is known to contribute to different biological processes such as appetite, sleeping, relaxation, hormone regulation, immunity, pains and inflammation responses. The interaction of cannabidoid in the endocannabinoid system assists homeostasis or the regulation of balance in the body.

According to scientific studies, the human body has 2 prime receptors of cannabinoids, these are known as CB1 and CB2. They are found within the cells of our body. Imagine million tiny cannabinoid receptor sites in the central nervous system and brain (CB1) while the rest are found in the immune system (CB2). These receptors interact through the neural communication process.

What is interesting to note is that the human body does not simply rely on cannabinoids produced by plants (phytocannabinoids). Mammals, especially humans, are capable of producing natural cannabinoids – the 2-AG and Anandamite. These two natural compounds which help the body control neural communication and mediate various cellular functions.

This vital information clearly showed that endocannabinoid system (ECS) is a very functional and essential regulatory system.

Medical Benefits of CBD

Many people from various parts of the world are starting to turn to the use of CBD to help cure their different health concerns.

Recent studies indicated that CBD contains anti-inflammatory, anti-anxiety and analgesic properties minus THC's psychoactive effects. To help you better understand this, below are the known benefits you can derive from the use of CBD:

CBD is associated with Adenosine receptor site activation. Cannabidoid can trigger the abundant release of glutamate neurotransmitters and dopamine. Glutamate is connected to cognition, memory formation, learning and excitatory signals. Dopamine is popularly known to aid in various processes including motor control, motivation, reward mechanism and cognition.

CBD is also known as pleitropic drug which can effectively pass through various molecular pathways.

It also inhibits the potential binding action of different receptors like the G-coupled proteins receptor.

CBD is greatly involved in 5-Ht1A serotonin receptor stimulation which provides anti-depressant effects. This receptor is directly involved with anxiety, appetite, nausea, pain perception and addiction.

CBD inhibits GPR55 signalling which remarkably reduces bone reabsorption, modulating the bone density, blood pressure control and hinders the proliferation of cancer cells.

CBD is utilized as anti-cancer treatment. When peroxisome proliferator activated receptors (PPAR) are fully activated in gamma level, they can induce significant regression of tumors in lung cancer cells. PPAR receptors are usually located on cell nucleus surfaces.

CBD can effectively stop cervical cancer cells from spreading. It decreases the ability of the tumor or cancer cells to produce energy which eventually weakens them and leads to the cells' natural death.

CBD-induced treatment assists lymphokine-activated killer (LAK) cells to overpower and kill debilitating cancer cells. It kills tumor cells found in colon cancer and leukemia. It decreases glioma cell invasion and growth. It is being studied as potential combination therapy for prostate and breast cancers.

CBD is eyed as potential remedy to treat Alzheimer's disease. The process involves hindering the development of PPAR-gamma amyloid-beta plaque. This molecule is considered the key link to the early stages of this disease.

CBD can benefit diabetics. PPAR receptors regulate insulin sensitivity, lipid uptake, energy homeostasis and metabolic functions. In a controlled experiment using non-obese mice, the onset of diabetes was prevented. Researchers explained that cannabidiol did not have a direct effect on glucose levels, however, it actively blocked splenocytes to produce IL-12, a type of cytokine which plays big role in different autoimmune diseases.

CBD can potentially alleviate the symptoms of epilepsy. It also controls the intensity and frequency of seizures.

However, thorough research is still being done to gain more understanding regarding this matter.

CBD can treat neuropsychiatric disorders which are also linked to epilepsy. This includes neuronal injury, psychiatric diseases and neurodegeneration. It can prevent toxicity which affects brain's radical oxygen species (ROS) and neurotransmitter glutamate which effectively prevent the death of brain cells. It can also protect the brain from the danger of ischemia.

CBD can control the development of Prion. Prions are types of proteins in the body which can bring neurogenerative diseases including Mad Cow and Creutzfeldt-Jakob. In 2007, the Journal of Neuroscience published the result of studies documenting the ability of CBD to stop the accumulation and formation of prions.

CBD is a possible cure for schizophrenia. German researchers conducted a controlled study among 42 patients in 2012. They used CBD and Amisulpride, a potent antipsychotic drug used for schizophrenic attacks. Both showed effectiveness, but with significant side effects. However, those who made use of CBD experienced far shorter post-treatment side effects when compared to others. The result of this study was published in Translational Psychiatry.

CBD is a potential treatment for Crohn's Disease. The anti-inflammatory components of cannabis can bring relief for bowel diseases including Crohn's Disease. Studies show that the CBD and THC compounds of cannabis can effectively interact and controls gut functions.

CBD can reduce effects of multiple sclerosis. Using cell culture and controlled animal models, the Cajal Institute scientists used CBD to find its effect to MS. The result showed positive effects. First, it reversed the inflammatory responses of the body. Second, it acted as a strong protection against the effects of the disease.

Other benefits include:

- *Natural Pain Reliever*

  CBD is a natural cure to lower mild to chronic pain. The non-psychoactive compounds it contains are being studied as a potential new treatment to ease chronic pain. Today, it is also utilized to help treat fibromyalgia and multiple sclerosis.

A 2011 experimental study which used CBD to treat fibromyalgia resulted to a promising result. Half of 56 participants were given CBD while the other half were given traditional anti-inflammatory drugs like corticosteroids and opioid. Those who used CBD induced treatment showed reduced pains and symptoms while those who used traditional cure continued experiencing discomfort.

- *Prevents and Controls Inflammation*

  Cannabidiol (CBD) decreases the growth and migration of neutrophils which trigger inflammation in the body. It also reduces B-cells chemokines production of macrophage inflammatory protein-1 alpha (MIP-1 alpha) and macrophage inflammatory protein-1 beta (MIP-1 beta).

  This ability of CBD makes it a potential therapeutic agent against various inflammatory disorders and pains.

- *Aids Drug and Smoking Withdrawal Symptoms*

  CBD is a potential treatment to assist people who seriously want to quit smoking. A pilot study where smokers were given inhalers with CBD compounds resulted to lesser cravings for nicotine. The participants would simply need to take a puff whenever they feel urge to smoke cigarette. It brought about a 40% drop of their cigarette consumption and eased the symptoms associated with the withdrawal process. The result of this experiment was published in *Addictive Behaviors*.

  Another experiment was conducted to discover the CBD effect to those addicted to opioid substances. The positive result was published in *Neurotherapeutics*.

- *Alleviates symptoms of anxiety disorders*

  It can be a potential cure for generalized anxiety disorder (GAD), post-traumatic stress disorder (PTSD), social anxiety, panic disorder and obsessive-compulsive disorder (OCD), as well as mild-to-severe cases of depression. CBD-induced treatment calms the patient and brings stable mental state.

Cannabinoids receptors in the brain are located in the area which regulates emotional behavior and responses, irritability, stress, fear, moods, sleep and "cravings". This part of the brain is comprised of the periaquenductal gray (PAG) of middle brain, hippocampus, prefrontal cortex, nucleus accumbens and amygdala. With presence of cannabidiol (CBD), the "fight or flight" stress sensation is triggered.

CBD treatment didn't show adverse effects when used for the above-mentioned disorders, a significant improvement compared to commercially-available medications.

- *Aids in curing insomnia*

Cannabis is a natural herb which can bring about a more relaxed stated and help people drift into easeful sleep. CBD-heavy strains treatment creates feelings of tiredness, one of its more positive side effects when it comes to insomnia.

Unlike sleeping pills, the good thing about the CBD treatment is that it is non-habit forming.

- *Heals Acne*

   This is also a potential cure for acne vulgaris. Acne is commonly caused by overworked sebaceous body glands or an inflammation inside the body. CBD treatment lowers sebum production and reduces inflammation. Cannabidiol acts like an anti-inflammatory and sebostatic agent which effectively inhibits lipid synthesis.

In summary, CBD is:

- anticonvulsant – it suppresses seizures

- antiemetic – reduces and alleviates vomiting or nausea

- anti-inflammatory – fights inflammatory issues

- antipsychotic – combats psychosis

- anti-cancer/anti-tumor - combats proliferation of cancer and tumor cells

- anti-depressant / anxiolytic – eliminates depression and anxiety symptoms

- antioxidants- fights various neurodegenerative problems

Possible Health Risks and Side Effects of CBD

The safety when using CBD is the primary concern of most people. Naturally, many studies have looked into this matter thoroughly and found that it is relatively safe for most people to use—of course, this also depends on any existing allergies that they might have, along with conditions that might not work well with the effects of CBD.

As for the basics, there were no significant side effects on the central nervous system nor did it cause any mood swings for people who used it continuously.

The most common side effect, however, is tiredness and feelings of fatigue. Other effects that some users have experienced also include: changes in weight, appetite, mild case of diarrhea or gastrointestinal discomfort, sleeping difficulty, dizziness and dry mouth. Again, this does not happen to everyone—only a select few.

Stopping the use of CBD oil too quickly does bring about certain effects as call, many of which are similar to nicotine withdrawal symptoms. This includes: nausea, dizziness, irritability and fogginess. It is best to lower the dose and talk to your doctor to assist you during this period.

Studies are still being conducted if it is safe to use CBD as treatment for children.

CHAPTER 4

HOW CBD WORKS IN THE BODY

You may wonder how cannabidoid enters the human cell and effectively binds to receptors. The process is intricate, yet efficient.

Cannabidoid passes through cell membranes and attaches itself to Fatty Acid Binding Proteins. This particular protein travels with lipid molecules and penetrates the interior of the cells. Interestingly, the same protein is responsible for Tetrahydrocannabinol (THC) transport, including the marijuana-like molecules produced by the brain – 2 AG and the Endocanabinoids Ananamide.

Once CBD is inside the cells, the fatty acid amide hydrolase (FAAH) begins breaking down the metabolic enzyme called Anandamide. FAAH is a vital component of the molecular life cycle of the cell.

The Endocannabinoid system and cannabinoids

The cannabinoids main target is the Endocannabinoid system or ECS. It is found in the central nervous system and in the brain. All mammals have this system in their bodies. ECS is the structural, molecular system which controls the body's reaction to normal psychological processes. This system in the body was first discovered in the late 1980s, and quickly became the subject of study because of its vital role in regulating homeostasis (general condition of balance). It corrects and mediates neural responses to help the body maintain its normal balance.

It is a signaling system which manages and controls the body's response to pain, sleep, hunger, stress, blood pressure, circadian rhythms, body temperature, moods, memory, fertility, metabolism, intestinal vitality, bone density and other vital functions. The Endocannabinoid system responds to natural endogenous cannabinoids which are manufactured by the body. The system can be manipulated to react to externally-induced cannabinoids to cure medical ailments—hence the effectiveness of CBD supplements.

Receptors of Endocannabinoid System and CBD

The Endocannabinoid system has millions of tiny receptor sites in almost all areas of the body. However, it only has two 2 main receptors which work to bind cannabinoids - CB1 and CB2.

CB1 receptors are found in the central nervous system and in the brain while **CB2** receptors are located in the immune system. They interact and work together through neural communication. The body's natural Endocannabinoids, the 2-AG and Anandamide control this cellular communication.

However, cannabidiol (CBD) from the cannabis hemp plant does not fit CB1 and CB2. *So how does it work when it enters the body?* CBD stimulates the receptor activities without binding itself to them. The result changes the cellular responses and can be systemic since CB1 and CB2 receptors are all over the body.

If THC is present in the system, CBD presence will counteract the known psychoactive effect of the compound on CB1 receptors.

Cytochrome P-450 System and CBD

Cannabidiol's ability to cure various illnesses can be done by manipulating the Endocannabinoid system. It is important for people to understand that CBD can be dangerous if improperly administered. CBD can inhibit the ability of *Cytochrome P-450 system* to metabolize medication for certain types of diseases. Cytochrome P-450 is a system found in the liver and is responsible for breaking down 90% of the drugs you take. This system has over 50 types of enzymes which process and flushes out toxins.

CBD presence in the system does prolong the processing of drugs and its effect on the body. This may also cause higher doses of drugs in the system, and if you're not careful, this can lead to an overdose or other adverse side-effects. It is vital to make dosage adjustments if you are taking both your medication drug and CBD.

Here are some of the drugs that utilize Cytochrome P-450 system which interact with cannabidiol (CBD):

- Antihistamines

- Antibiotics

- Steroids

- Anesthetics

- Benzodiazepines

- Calcium channel blockers

- Anti-psychotics

- Anti-depressants

- Anti-arrythmics

- Anti-epileptics

- Prokinetics

- Immune modulators

- Beta blockers

- HIV antivirals

- HMG CoA reductase inhibitors

- Sulfonylureas

- Angiotension II blockers

- Oral hypoglycemic agents

- PPIs

- NSAIDs

It is vital to consult your doctor before taking CBD dietary supplements so they can adjust the dosage for your other medications. While you are there, ask him to test your Cytochrome P-450 system to make sure that it is functioning excellently and metabolizing your medications as it should.

Other Effects of CBD

Cannabidiol can also affect the other functions of our bodies.

One of them is binding itself to G-protein coupled receptors (TRPV-1). This receptor regulates body inflammation, perceptions of pains and mediating body temperature.

It activates the receptors that stimulate serotonin.

And finally, its potent power inhibits the ID-1 gene which is responsible for the formation of aggressive types of cancers in brain, breast, pancreas, lungs and ovaries.

The Entourage Effect

In alternative medicine, the whole plant is utilized for medicinal use to gain its optimum benefits. Note that its plant form is known to be more effective for treating various medical conditions when compared to synthetic forms of substance.

The whole and cooperative effects of cannabinoids including terpenoids and flavonoids were observed by cannabis science pioneer Dr. Raphael Mechoulam and his team. They called it the "entourage effect."

"Entourage effect" is a phenomenon produced by the interaction of natural plant components with the body to bring more potent effects for treating a disease. The combined power of multiple and natural

compounds has a multiplying effect which benefits the body. Every compound can amplify the ability of other compounds to bring over-all treatment of diseases.

Cannabis for instance has many active compounds which include the most popular- the cannabidiol (CBD) and the tetrahyrocannabinol (THC). These various forms of compounds in cannabis work together and alleviate negative symptoms. CBD can both modulate and neutralize THC effects on the body. When a person takes marijuana which contains high-amount of THC, this makes them feel "high". On the other hand, the hemp plant, which contains more cannabidiol (CBD), would instead bring relief to the body minus the psychoactive effect. Specially-bred cannabis marijuana has almost equal amounts of CBD and THC, and can be effectively used to alleviate pain and various other symptoms.

Terpene is another botanical component which is known to contain volatile molecules which easily evaporate. There are about 200 terpenes or terpenoids in cannabis plants although only few contain substantial amounts to be note-worthy, this includes: sesquiterpenes, diterpenes and monoterpenes. They contain isoprene or repeating 5-carbon molecule units.

One popular type of sesquitere is the beta-caryophyllene. It is the oil found in black pepper, oregano, several cannabis strains and many green, leafy vegetables. It can directly adhere or bind itself to CB2 or the peripheral cannabinoid receptors. This component helps protect the gastrointestinal tract and can also treat certain types of ulcer. It also offers potential promise as treatment for auto-immune disorders and inflammatory issues. The ability of beta-caryophyllene to easily bind itself to CB2 receptors makes it a "dietary cannabinoid."

The interaction of cannabinoids and terpenoids create potent synergy that kills active respiratory pathogens including the antibiotic-resistant MRSA bacteria. It also enhances cortical activity, increases blood circulation, and treats inflammation, anxiety, depression, cancer, epilepsy, addiction, pain, bacterial and fungal infections.

So why not use the entire plant?

Despite the above-mentioned benefits of using the whole plant, it is not feasible in many places, particularly in the US, because of the following reasons:

1. The botanical extracts' potency is not consistent due to weather and environmental conditions.

2. Because of the insufficient understanding of its components that bring therapeutic effects to the body, botanical products are not standardized.

3. The Food and Drug Administration (FDA) is not closely monitoring herbal products which can result to poor quality control. This can bring adulterated, contaminated, unsafe and less effective botanical products.

However, there are ongoing studies with the purpose of shedding more light on the capability of using whole plants to cure diseases and harnessing their full therapeutic potency.

The public become more aware of this *"entourage effect"* when Dr. Sanjay Gupta, a neurosurgeon and media personality wrote about it being effective to reduce spasms and pain of Multiple Sclerosis instead of medication containing single compound.

Clinical Endocannabinoid Deficiency Syndrome (CEDS)

CEDS is the medical term for one group of diseases which includes: fibromyalgia, irritable bowel syndrome and migraine. According to various scientists and medical experts, these illnesses are caused by low endocannabinoid level in the body.

The level of endocannabinoids can affect the proper functioning of some body systems. Very low endocannabinoid level brings active CEDS symptoms. One significant study regarding CEDS found that Anandamide receptors are directly affected by insufficient amount of endocannabinoids in the body. These receptors are closely linked to periaqueductal gray matter otherwise known as "migraine generator" of the human brain. This endocannabinoid deficiency can trigger symptoms of migraine and other conditions under CEDS. Increased and sufficient level stops adverse gastrointestinal, peripheral and spinal actions.

To overcome this condition, you would need to increase your Omega-3 fatty acid intake. This will also increase the production of natural endogenous cannabinoids. It also heals and facilitates growth of your CB1 receptors.

Taking CBD or cannabidiol to supplement the endogenous cannabinoids of the body helps to correct the deficiency. It leads to more active and efficient endocannabinoid system.

CHAPTER 5

CBD HEMP OIL

One of the fastest-growing products in the oil industry is the Cannabidiol hemp oil (CBD hemp oil). It has become a highly-demanded oil in more than 40 countries and 50 states of United States.

Cannabidiol hemp oil became widely sought after a highly-publicized media exposure. It has taken the general public by storm after Dr. Sanjay Gupta presented a television special documentary called "Weed" in CNN. He investigated and documented the ability of cannabidoid to treat children suffering from epilepsy.

The initial purpose is to view it as medicine for critically-ill patients, but the general public's interest kept on growing and more studies have since been made into just how beneficial it can be for treating different illnesses as well as for boosting a person's overall health. There was an instant demand and people were looking for place where they could buy CBD hemp oil. Grocery stores, doctor's clinics and medical marijuana dispensaries started displaying CBD hemp oil. Purchasing the product is easy and does not require medical card.

The oil is extracted from seeds and stalk of industrial hemp plant. It contains large quantity of CBD or cannabidiol compounds. However, the extraction process must also ensure that it produces highly-concentrated CBD oil and doesn't change it in any way. The oil is also abundant with other nutrients like vitamins, amino acids, Omega-3 fatty acids, chlorophyll, terpenes, and phytocannabinoids such as cannabidivarian (CBCV), canabicromene (CBD), cannabinol (CBN) and cannabigerol (CBG).

Full-Spectrum Hemp Oil

Full-spectrum refers to a hemp oil that is pure and concentrated. It contains the same amount and quality of compounds and cannabinoids of the source plant. Unlike synthetic products, this type of hemp oil has a dozen forms of cannabinoids plus vitamins, minerals, protein, fatty acids, chlorophyll, fiber, terpenes and flavonoids.

Cannabinoids

Full spectrum hemp oil contains abundant supply of cannabidiol (CBD). It amounts to more than 90% of total cannabinoids. Hemp oil has cannabinoid cannabidiolic acid (CBDa) which turns into CBD compound during heating process or decarboxylation. Aside from CBD, full-spectrum hemp oil has other major forms of cannabinoids such as tetrahydrocannabinol (THC), cannabinol (CBN) and cannabigerol (CBG).

Vitamins and Minerals

Full-spectrum hemp oil has great quantity of essential vitamins A, C, E and B-complex vitamins (niacin, riboflavin and thiamine). It is also a good source of beta-carotene and other forms of vitamins which are not abundantly available in daily diets.

Minerals such as iron, zinc, calcium, magnesium, potassium and phosphorous can be found from full-spectrum hemp oil. These minerals are vital for metabolic processes, bodily functions, nerve functions, building strong bones, and healthy skin, skin and blood circulation.

Essential Proteins and Fats

Protein is the building block of muscles. It repairs tissues and cells. Hemp oil contains 9 essential amino acids and 11 others which are all important for body functions.

Fatty acids are important compounds to sustain cardiovascular health and excellent heart condition. Full-spectrum hemp oil has essential fatty acids like Omega-3 and Omega-6.

CBD Hemp Oil versus Hemp Oil

Be mindful that CBD hemp oil is different from organic hemp oil that is commercially available in grocery stores.

Hemp oil or hempseed oil does not have cannabidiol. However, it contains vitamins, minerals and other nutrients. It is produced by pressing the seeds of hemp. Unrefined and cold-pressed hemp oil has nutty flavor and has a dark green to light green color. The darker the color, the grassier the taste. It is rich in omega-3 to omega-6 fatty acids. The nutritional value is about 1:3 which matches the body's requirement.

Refined hemp oil is colorless with little flavor. It does not have natural nutrients such as vitamins and lacks antioxidant properties. The refined form is usually utilized as ingredients for body care essentials such as soaps and shampoos. It is also used in detergents. Industrial hemp oil is commonly used for plastics, lubricants, fuel, paints and inks. It has a subject of studies as potential feedstock to produce biodiesel in large-scale level.

Hempseed oil comes from Cannabis sativa varieties which do not have high components of tetrahydrocannabinol (THC). There is no THC element in hempseed. The traces that are found present in hemp oil can be due to adherence of plant matter to seed surface when it is manufactured. In Canada, the manufacturers successfully lowered THC content when they started using more modern production methods back in 1998. Sampling showed 4ppm or parts per million (4 mg.kg.) which is below the 10 ppm detection limit. Other countries in Europe impose 5ppm to none detection limit.

On the other hand, CBD hemp oil is a botanical, highly-concentrated and pure form of cannabidiol. It is extracted from the stalks, leaves and flowers. It supports general health and well-being. It is also non-addictive and safe to use. Its potency to bring therapeutic benefits is now widely-known. Hemp CBD dietary supplements are regulated by the FDA.

Methods of CBD Hemp Oil Extraction

There are three methods to extract this valuable oil from hemp plants.

1. Oil Method – It is the most popular way to produce oil from industrial hemp. It uses carrier oils, such as olive oil, for the process. The combined power of CBD hemp oil and carrier oil brings greater benefits to users. It also prevents unwanted residues and guarantees safety.

2. CO_2 Method – The procedure involves pushing CO_2 out of hemp at high pressure levels and low temperature. The process

results to a pure form of CBD. It is considered the safest and the best way to extract the oil because it removes unwanted substances like chlorophyll and does not leave unsafe residues. It also produces a cleaner taste, but the process is expensive.

This process requires equipment that can force the cannabinoid solution and CO2 to separate from each other. During this, the cannabinoids would go to different chambers than the CO2. Manufacturers like this process because it enables them to "customize" the resulting product.

3. Ethanol Method – This process of oil extraction involves the use of high-grain alcohol which can destroy the natural oils elements.

Rick Simpson was the originator of using alcohol to extract an "original" or purer type of CBD oil. He soaked hemp material in a solvent and after a while, it produced liquid which is full of cannabidoids. He then evaporated the solvent to leave only the essential liquid.

His method was copied and used by large-scale manufacturers to produce commercially-available CBD hemp oil products. The alcohol solution that is left behind is put through "Roto-Vap" which separates ethanol from the oil. The alcohol goes to another chamber instead of evaporating and the machine stores it for future use. The oil that is left is ready for users' consumption.

How to produce your own CBD

You can produce your own CBD or cannabidoids at home using simple and safe techniques. You do not need special skills or expensive equipment to make your own oil.

What you need

- 30 grams of ground hemp buds (60-100 ground of ground, dried trim)

- 4l grain alcohol (any high-proof and food-safe alcohol) Grain alcohol is the best option because it doesn't leave any unpleasant and harmful residue. It is an excellent solvent for extracting small batches of cannabis oil.

- ceramic (or glass) mixing bowl

- fine strainer (sieve, cheesecloth, nylon stocking)

- double boiler (or set of 2 pots/saucepans with space in between when they are stacked together)

- catchment container

- silicon spatula

- plastic syringe

- wooden spoon

- funnel

Procedure

- Start by setting up your tools.

- Place the hemp material in the mixing bowl, then put grain alcohol and stir the solution for 3-5 minutes using wooden spoon.

- Mix thoroughly to expel resin. Make sure that your mixing bowl is large enough to contain the plant material and solvent.

- Next, filter the solution into the drainer then collect the initial raw extraction and placed it in the catchment container. Squeeze the liquid.

- Transfer the collected liquid to the double burner and heat it. Wait until it bubbles. Allow the alcohol to evaporate. Keep the temperature at minimal level. You can also turn it on and off to keep the gentle bubbling of the solution for 15-30 minutes.

- Stir regularly. Do not allow the solution to be too hot. When you see alcohol evaporating, carefully mix the liquid using the silicon spatula.

- Your solution is ready. Transfer the oil to a bottle or containers before it becomes thick. Use a plastic syringe or pour the concentrated CBD oil to small, airtight and dark dosage bottles.

*While still warm, dilute the concentrated extract with coconut oil, olive oil or vegetable oil of your choice to make excellent ointment for topical use.

CHAPTER 6

DIFFERENT TYPES OF CBD HEMP OIL

CBD and THC act on different enzymes and receptors. Using CBD infused products can effectively counteract the effects of THC like over-excitability and paranoia. It is 100% non-psychoactive, non-addictive and safe.

Hemp oil products can be purchased legally in any part of America and other countries across the globe including: Argentina, Austria, Belgium, Belize, Brazil, Bulgaria, Canada, Chile, China, Colombia, Costa Rica, Croatia, Cyprus, Czech Republic, Denmark, England, Estonia, Finland, France, Georgia, Germany, Greece, Guam, Guatemala, Hong Kong, Hungary, Iceland, India, Ireland, Italy, Latvia, Lithuania, Luxembourg, Malta, Netherlands, Netherlands Antilles, Northern Ireland, Norway, Paraguay, Peru, Poland, Portugal, Puerto Rico, Romania, Russia, Scotland, Slovak

Republic, Slovenia, South Africa, Sweden, Switzerland, U.S. Virgin Islands, United Kingdom, Uruguay and Wales.

There are various forms and concentrations of CBD. These include liquid hemp oil, oil in capsules, hemp oil in thick paste form, sprays or sublingual tincture drops, CBD vaporizers (vapes), concentrates, salves for topical application and edibles (gum or candy).

When taken orally, it is necessary to hold the solution under your tongue to allow direct absorption before swallowing it. This step is important because the digestive system can break the CBD down once it reaches the stomach.

CBD hemp oil, when taken at lower dosages, relaxes and calms the body.

Tinctures

Tincture is a liquid extract intended for oral use. The exact amount of CBD solution is measured by the product's dropper top. It is the most common form of CBD laden product. It is the purest application since manufacturers do not use separation methods to extract the oil. There are brands which have a little flavor which is helpful for consumers who do like a little taste during consumption.

It is considered to be the most effective way to gain the benefits of CBD. Its ability to bring precise dosages ensures optimum benefit. It is also very easy to increase or decrease the quantity you take.

You can also opt to mix the CBD tincture with your favorite drink while on the go. The recommended dose is from 100mg-1000mg. It is vital to know your needs or start slow and gradually increase the dosage to find the strength you need. There are many flavors available in the market today. CBD tinctures are now flavored with vanilla, cinnamon, peppermint and many more. Others have sweeteners to make them tastier.

The downside of using tinctures is messiness if you spill some of it during usage but this is just a minor issue.

How to apply

Shake the solution well. Separation of oil with the other elements of the product is natural when it is not used. Shaking it blends all the helpful ingredients of the solution and neutralizes the strong taste.

Use the dropper top and fill the pipette then dispense 2 drops of oil under your tongue. Swish it around your mouth or let it sit for 30-90 seconds to allow your system to fully absorb the oil.

If the taste is too strong for you, drink juice or apple cider to neutralize the hempy flavor as you ingest it. Repeat when needed throughout the whole day.

Concentrates or Oil Form

This form is the most popular among users who want a more potent form of CBD. This contains high-dosages of cannabidiol. Typically, 10 times stronger compared to other types. It is more convenient to use. CBD concentrates have little to no flavor for those who do not want the bland taste of oil.

The downside is its inability to be flavored. It can be a big deal for people who cannot take natural flavors and are unable to swallow down the oil. For beginners, concentrates can be a little shocking because their shapes are like syringes.

How to apply

Like tincture, placing it under the tongue and ingesting it slowly is the way to consume it.

Sprays

This is the weakest form of CBD when it comes to concentration. The typical CBD concentration usually amounts anywhere from 1-3 mg. It is difficult to measure the right dosage because spray is a little bit inconsistent.

One of the advantages of using spray is convenience and it can be used whenever needed. It is easier to spray CBD oil into the mouth compared to using concentrate or tincture if you are on a travel.

How to apply

Spray one dosage CBD oil into your mouth. The right dosage should be on the bottle label. The typical instruction is 2-3 sprays daily or as needed.

Capsules

Taking in CBD oil in capsule form is the easiest method if you're using it as a daily supplement. It is usually packaged in dissolvable capsules with high CBD concentration. It is odorless and tasteless. It works well with other supplements like vitamins or minerals. Each package contains 2-60 capsules. It makes measuring or tracking down your daily dosage easier. When in doubt, it is easy to know if you are able to take your daily dose by counting the remaining capsules.

One downside of CBD capsule is when you want to up your dosage by a bit but you don't' want to swallow 2 capsules. One way to address this concern is to add other forms of CBD product such as tincture to adjust your serving size every day.

How to apply

Take one capsule a day or as needed.

Topical

Many topical brands in the market now are laden with CBD. This includes: lip balms, creams lotions and salves. Products with CBD help in anti-aging, inflammation, cancer treatment, chronic pain, psoriasis and acne. The topical products have unique usability which includes targeting specific areas of inflammation or stiffness in the body. Topical CBD products are easily-absorbed and can be used to directly alleviate pain and discomfort of the body zones.

When selecting topical products, check the following keywords which indicate that it uses CBD-encapsulation: ***micellization and nano technology***. These indicators are proof that the product can penetrate easily through the skin's dermal layer and makes CBD work not just on the outer skin, but also deep within.

However, because topical products by skin absorption, it does have a tendency to work slower compared to other forms of CBD products. The products –lotions, balms and creams are also more expensive because they are infused with high-quality ingredients aside from cannabidiol.

How to apply

Like any other topical body care products, apply it generously to affected area of the body. Use it as often as necessary.

Vaporizers

Smoking CBD or vaporizing CBD oil helps the user adjust the dosage that's right for them. Think of it as being very similar to an e-cigarette or e-pen. The CBD oil is heated up into a vapor before it can be inhaled. The vaporizing methods works fast and is also safe for the oral tract because. Note that vaporizers do not produce smoke.

When purchasing vaporizers, you will receive two products – the vaporizer and CBD cartridges which contain the oil. Vaporizes are convenient, handy, lightweight and a stylish form of using CBD.

It has lesser drawback compared to taking CBD products orally. Concentrates, tinctures and capsules take a longer period to be absorbed which brings delayed effect.

How to apply

You need vaporizer, inhaler, e-cigarette or vape pen. Add appropriate amount of CBD hemp oil to your device, heat and inhale.

Edibles

Nowadays, CBD can be excellently lumped into variety of edibles.

Chocolate bar - One of the most popular edible forms is a CBD laden bar of chocolate. It offers many great benefits and is also very easy to consume. It also masks the distinct hempy taste. Chocolate bars allows you to effectively control the dosage you take. It is a more discreet way of taking CBD.

Most CBD chocolate bars are infused with about 10mg of hemp oil. If this is your desired amount, you can consume it at once or take smaller bites throughout the day. There are also variety of flavors – dark chocolate, mint dark chocolate, Raspberry Milk chocolate and more.

CBD Gums/Chews

There are gums or chews with CBD oil. These edible products promote instant calm. CBD can also be combined effectively with other elements like essential vitamins, caffeine and flavors to enhance the benefits of the product.

1 piece of gum/chew taken as necessary is recommended.

CBD Lozenges

Lozenges with CBD are refreshingly good because of their minty taste. Most brands offer sugar-free, gluten free, dairy free products and preservative-free for consumers who have special dietary needs.

It is easy to use lozenges. Just pop one into your mouth. It is best taken on an empty stomach. 1-2 lozenges a day is the recommended serving for optimum CBD absorption.

CBD Dab Oils or Wax

To produce wax, solvent is used during extraction process. Using vape pens, it is applied through dabbing. It instantly help with reducing chronic pain, inflammation and anxiety. It produces potent relief with just 2-3 strokes of vape pen.

Gel Pen

It gently soothes and offers lasting relief when applied to affected area of the body. Gel pens are perfect for patients who suffer from consistent chronic pains. It is safe to use and does not bring adverse side effects. It is also light to carry anywhere.

The best method of using this is to put an amount of gel to areas with superficial veins like temples, wrists or ankles (or any part where you can clearly see your veins). Gently press the pen's tip on the spot then spread the gel for maximum absorption. It usually works within 15-20 minutes upon application. If you are unsure of the appropriate amount that would work for you, can start with a small amount then increase it gradually to get the desired result you need.

Do not use if you are lactating or pregnant. For patients with chronic illness or taking regular medication, consult your doctor first to know if it is safe for you to use CBD gel pens.

Always keep the product in dry, cool place. Secure it away from pets and little children.

CBD Patches

Patches are infused with CBD are therapeutic. Most brands would contain 2.5mg of pure CBD and no

THC. You can use it at once or cut it to spread the dosage within the day. It is best for users with anxiety issues and fibromyalgia condition.

It works after 15-20 minutes. The sensation it brings is mild and does not interfere with regular daily tasks. After 45 to an hour, the curing sensation stops and leaves you feeling better. It brings physical and mental relief for the next hours.

CHAPTER 7

HOW TO USE CBD HEMP OIL

The prime source of CBD oil is hemp or industrial hemp. CBD oil is a natural, concentrated, non-psychoactive extract from hemp plant which contains low-THC and high-CBD components. At present, there are many brands, types and forms of CBD hemp oil that are available for both skin care and dietary needs.

Pure CBD hemp oil can also be taken directly as dietary or nutritional supplement. Its concentrated form can be used topically or infused into body and skin care products. The therapeutic and beauty benefits of CBD oil gave rise to various product forms – drops, capsules and chewing gum.

The many benefits of CBD hemp oil has certainly changed public opinion about it. The once-taboo herb is now more associated with supplemental nutrition values. The potential of cannabidiol hemp oil to address the nutritional needs of consumers brought it to public awareness. There were about 23,000 published studies in various medical journals giving information about the good benefits of cannabis oil and cannabinoids in human body without the "high" effect.

With increased interest in CBD hemp oil, it is important to understand how this oil can help the nutritional requirements of consumers.

Because there is no scientifically-proven and recommended dosing regimen, it is important to do it step-by-step. Begin at small dosage then gradually adjust the concentration to address your specific need. Every product has recommended daily serving which you can follow. However, it is best to do some studies regarding hemp oil so you would know how much dosage you need and how often.

Dietary Supplements

CBD hemp oil has variety of concentrated forms, ranging in amount anywhere from 1 mg/serving up to 80 mg/serving. The wide range of CBD concentration is helpful for those who want to maximize their usage to suit their purposes. All dietary supplements have clear instructions with suggested serving doses and the CBD amount per serving.

A little amount of CBD can greatly benefit a user. If it is your first time to use CBD dietary supplements, it is best to start with a low concentration then slowly increase the dosage along the way. You can also speak to your physician about what might be the right amount for you depending on what you're using for, as well as if you're taking other supplements at the moment.

Methods of CBD Hemp Oil Consumption

There are several factors that influence the impact of CBD on human health. It includes dosage, mode of consumption and symptoms of the medical trouble.

- Vape – It is the most convenient, efficient and safest way.

- Sublingual – It produces fast relief within few minutes.

- Topical – It the slowest and you need to apply uniform amount of CBD hemp oil to ensure optimum result.

- Orally – It takes about 30-60 minutes to feel the result. It is best taken on empty stomach.

- Add-on to food or drink – It help cure headaches and dysphoria. Although, it takes long time to feel the effect, it guarantees no adverse side effects.

What is The Standard Amount?

Many doctors, when asked for CBD supplement prescriptions are reluctant because there is no guiding prescription available. Pharmacology courses do not tackle CBD's proper dosage. Medical scientists are only beginning to develop dosing schedules for the medical use of hemp extracts and medical marijuana.

Different brands offer different standards of CBD dosage which can be very confusing for many people, especially for first time users.

CBDOilReview.org (COR) provided simple standard which you can consider. It recommends CBD serving of 25mg twice within the day. You can gradually increase your consumption by 25mg every 3-4 weeks. If side effects manifest during consumption, decrease the dosage.

General guidelines for CBD Hemp Oil Usage for Treatment:

- Chronic Pain

  2.5- 20 mg by mouth for 25 days

- Epilepsy

  200 – 300 mg by mouth every day for 4 ½ months

- Sleep Disorders/Insomia

  40-160 mg by mouth when needed

- Huntington's disease

  To ease movement problem, take 10 mg/kilogram by mouth every day for 1 ½ months

- Schizophrenia

  40- 1,280 mg by mouth every day for up to one month

- Multiple Sclerosis Symptoms

  2.5 -120 mg of CBD-THC combination by mouth every day from 2-15 weeks. Mouth spray containing the compounds is given to patients up to 8 weeks. A maximum of 48 sprays per day or 8 sprays every 3 hours is recommended to maximize the benefits.

- Glaucoma

  20-40 mg placed under tongue every day. More than 40 mg dosage is dangerous because it increases eye pressure.

There is no recorded case of lethal CBD dose. But, consumers must follow the instructions thoroughly to find the right dosage and maximize its effects. It is highly important to talk to your physician and get prescription from him before taking CBD supplements.

CHAPTER 8

GUIDE FOR BUYING CBD HEMP OIL

At this point in time, you may be wondering about where to buy and how to buy CBD hemp oil and other CBD products. In this chapter, we breakdown all the information you need to know.

Initially, you would need to consider the best CBD brand, the concentration of CBD, the type of CBD product and your particular purpose or need for the product. CBD products come in different forms, shapes and sizes. Comparing and distinguishing which among the almost similar products is best for you is necessary before making a final decision.

- *CBD Volume*

  Find out the amount of CBD in each product. Different brands and products offer varying CBD content. To find out the quantity, make sure that the product specifically refers to CBD and not the overall quantity of hemp oil.

CBD product is typically measured using two quantities – CBD quantity and Hemp Oil quantity (total volume of oil content). Always check for CBD quantity in the label.

- *CBD Concentration*

Concentration is another essential characteristic that you need to look for in CBD hemp oil product. This determines how much cannabidiol in the product. Amounts can vary anywhere from: normal strength to super-high CBD concentration or hundred percent pure natural concentration ranges.

CBD concentration would aid you in finding the right dosage you need to maximize the benefit. It is recommended for adult beginners to take small doses of about 1-3mg every day. Gradually, you can adjust the size of serving once the body becomes accustomed with the substance. You can double the amount the week after your first try or adjust the quantity to find the accurate quantity your body specifically needs. Because CBD does not have psychoactive effects, you can safely take optimal concentration to gain its benefits just like what multi-vitamins supplements do to the body.

- *Types of CBD products*

  CBD hemp oil is a versatile substance which can be effectively turned into different types of products – from capsules, tinctures, vaporizers and more. Whatever form it takes, the health benefits that it offers remain potent. However, different brands offer different concentrations, flavors and method of consumption (there are CBD hemp oils that are designed to be added to drinks or foods while others are produced for synergistic effects).

Other factors that you need to consider before buying CBD hemp oil are:

- *Manufacturer/Distributor Track Record*

  It is essential to do basic research first and look for a company that has a reliable track record. Read reviews regarding the company and find out users' comments about their experience with buying from the company. It is important to make sure that you purchase high-quality, effective and safe CBD hemp oil. Despite being a new industry in the market, there are already established brands out there that would be able to provide you with quality products.

- *Clear Labeling Design*

  It is vital to get a product that provides you with a proper label, one that outlines all the ingredients of the product. It must clearly show other essential details such as expected shelf life, standard serving size and proper storage method.

- *Avoidance of Health Claims*

  CBD hemp oil in United States is categorized under dietary supplements. Any company that claims its ability to cure any medical case is violating FDA's DSHEA rules and regulation.

Where to buy CBD Hemp Oil

The importation of CBD hemp oil and other dietary supplements that contains CBD is now legal. It is easy to purchase the product online in over 40 manufacturing countries around the world.

It is readily available for consumers who want to try the effectiveness of CBD in addressing different health concerns. CBD hemp oil products can be bought in online stores, medical marijuana dispensaries and in various wellness or natural products stores.

When buying CBD hemp oil, always check for quality and try to avoid low-priced brands. Do not be tempted by affordability, always focus on its quality even if it means you have to pay a little extra. CBD quality is measured by the quantity of the cannabidiol concentration that the product contains. The higher the concentration, the more potent its effects would be.

CHAPTER 9

IS CBD HEMP OIL GOOD FOR PETS?

According to scientific studies, all animals except insects produce endocabinnoids. The presence of endocabinnoid system in animal bodies helps them regulate their physiological responses. Like humans, there are receptors throughout their bodies that can be activated by inducing phytocannabinoids-- in particular cannabidoid (CBD. CBD can effectively cure the underlying symptoms of disease among animals in a more natural way.

So, is it safe to give your dog or pets?

The answer is yes. Based on research and experiments conducted by scientists, CBD also benefits animals. CBD was first mixed with edible canine treats and were given to animals who were suffering from pain, inflammation and cancer-related issues—this showed positive results. CBD can also be utilized for fatal ailments or palliative care.

Pets, especially dogs, who are suffering from severe arthritis or inoperable cancer experience muscle wasting and usually have no appetite. CBD can help with that as well. In using it, pet owners can also avoid the risk of damaging their pet's kidney and liver which happens due to constant use of synthetic medication.

CBD contains very low THC so it will not make your pet high. One common side effect of cannabidiol, however, is drowsiness which is not dangerous. Other rare side effects are mild vomiting and itchiness.

<u>Can it be used to treat chronic and acute conditions?</u>

CBD is beneficial to pets suffering from acute and chronic diseases. Chronic conditions include: aggression, compromised immune system, digestive issues, osteoarthritis and stress. There are also ongoing studies if cannabidiol can effectively treat different canine cancers, Type 1 diabetes and organ diseases.

Cannabidiol (CBD) treatments have also been found to be beneficial for treating acute ailments such as bone breakage, strains and sprains, torn ligaments and post-operative issues like stiffness, swelling and pain.

Pet owners who do not want to see their canine pets suffering are looking for ways to provide them with relief and ease the pain their beloved pets are feeling. CBD can help with this as well. Furthermore, it is known to soothe pet anxiety-- especially during veterinary visits, fear from thunderstorm, separation anxiety, social anxiety and traveling in cars. These vouched the ability of CBD to help canine pets and their owners.

Why are veterinarians cautious when prescribing CBD?

Despite the benefits of CBD induced treatment, it is not yet prescribed by most veterinarians. They refrain from endorsing cannabis plant extracts due to two reasons.

First: Issues with misinformation and pet owners using actual cannabis in treating their pets. These concerns are validated when recreational cannabis was legalized in different states including Colorado. Many dogs suffered from marijuana poisoning caused by large consumption of cannabis which contains high amounts of THC. Dogs would often suffer seizures then go into coma and eventually die.

Second: The lack of understanding and awareness of non-psychoactive cannabinoids like CBD. Many veterinarians still have a predominant view that cannabis is a toxic plant. Sad to say, there are still large numbers of vets who are unaware that cannabis has different strains and most of them do not produce psychoactive effects.

There is also a clout of doubt that many veterinarians are resisting CBD induced treatments because this may affect the multi-billion dollar pet medication industry. As of 2013, the Federal Trade Commission reported a $ 7.6 billion sales and expected to balloon to $10.2 billion dollars in 2018.

Does CBD work fast even for pets?

Cannabidiol is a botanical or herbal drug which does not bring instant effects. It usually takes two hours to be fully ingested an absorbed to their system. However, it can arrest pain within few minutes but you will need to wait longer for inflammation and other underlying symptoms to heal.

Is CBD metabolism among dogs similar to humans?

The answer is no. Dogs metabolize cannabidiol in different way. Do you remember the anandamide and 2-AG compounds? These two natural chemicals are produced by the human body and are also present in canines as well. These 2 chemicals activate and trigger CB1 and CB2 receptors in canines. CBD tend to bind these 2 receptors for a longer period thus creating long-lasting therapeutic benefits for dogs without causing any toxic effect.

During intravenous infusions conducted to see the effect of cannabidiol in canines, there was a rapid response which is followed with 9-hour terminal half-life. It caused low oral bioavailability of about 13-19%. This also helps eliminate systemic toxicity among dogs. After the effects wane, the CBD is metabolized by the dog's liver and flushes it out of the body naturally. This can be the reason of immediate and long-lasting effects of CBD to diseased animals.

So what do the different studies reveal?

Studies supporting cannabinoid use among for animals showed that CBD was able to improve their mobility. It also improved their pet's appetite and successfully reduced their tendency to rely on traditional synthetic veterinary drugs. Most canines actually develop an intolerance to these drugs.

Another study showed that cannabinoids can effectively prevent inflammatory allergic problems, skin diseases and immune-mediated health issues in pets. CBD also has higher level of anti-epileptic and anticonvulsant properties compared to conventional drugs that are used to treat these conditions.

Other studies show that the following medical conditions were successfully relieved using edible CBD treats – pain, inflammation, nausea or vomiting, nervous system problems, anxiety, tumors, convulsions, seizures, digestive system disorders, phobias and skin problems.

CBD is also beneficial for canines suffering from osteoarthritis (OA) that causes neuropathic pain.

What other animals can benefit from cannabidoid (CBD)?

Aside from dogs, the other mammal with an endocannabinoid system is the mice. Invertebrate and vertebrate species like cats, chicken, turtles, sea urchin and fish also have cannabinoid receptors that respond to phytocannabinoids.

However, there are distinct differences in the cannabinoid systems of these species. Rodents like mice and rats have cannabinoid receptors that are mostly located along the brain's cerebellum and basal ganglia. These areas control their body movements and coordination. Humans, in comparison, have a lower concentration of receptors in these areas.

One of the most common neurological disorders among dogs is epilepsy. Studies reveal that epileptic dogs have high level of endocannabidoids in their endocannabinoid system. This is because these compounds are attempting to combat seizures caused by the disease. Another answer is the possibility that seizures damaged the normal functioning of the endocannabinoid system and caused higher levels of endocannabinoid production in their bodies.

<u>What is the proper dosage for dogs?</u>

Different types of health conditions among dogs need different dosages. It is best to start with a low dosage of CBD hemp oil then gradually adjust to the recommended amount. This way can help your dog's body gets accustomed with its effects.

One recommended method is giving 1 drop per 10 pounds of your dog's weight every day for about one week. Then, give it 1 drop twice a day during the second week until you manage to find the proper dosage that gives relief and cures the illness of your dog minus the side effects.

If they aren't showing any side effects, you can continue increasing the amount of CBD oil every 4-5 days until such time you clearly see the therapeutic benefits of cannabidiol (CBD). When there is any presence of side effects such as vomiting, disorientation, excessive sedation and hyperactivity, stop CBD treatment and allow them to pass. After some time, begin again with lower dose.

If you are using CBD treats like cookies, be sure not to exceed the maximum recommended amount in the instruction. A quarter of a piece at the beginning is best for your pets. Avoid handing CBD treats like regular food treats. Store them in place where your pets cannot easily access them.

Things to remember when purchasing CBD treats for your dogs:

First, use products that are especially formulated for the type of pet you have.

Second, choose which form of CBD you think will benefit your pets the most. CBD products come in tincture or oil form and food treats. Tinctures are the most common method to administer CBD oil to your dog. Putting the oil directly into your pet's mouth can be messy so you can choose to use treats.

Third, many online stores are selling CBD products for pets. To make sure that you are getting a product that's legitimate, you can choose to buy directly from manufacturers or their authorized stores.

CONCLUSION

Understanding how cannabidiol or CBD works to help sustain health and freedom from chronic to acute diseases is empowering. It helps consumers find answers to some of the most common health concerns which are often overlooked. Learning that the answer is simple and accessible makes it easy for everyone to find natural medications which are not only safe, but also effective in combating the symptoms of illnesses that can be debilitating as time goes on.

Pure botanical phytocannabinoids including CBD have proven their health benefits and has since become the subject of many studies. This injected life back into the hemp industry into the market, something that benefits not just its users, but the people who grow them as well.

With more published works being released and reflecting positive views on this beneficial plant, people are learning that it isn't something that's wholly bad—that there is a very distinct difference between the marijuana and hemp plant. A difference that they could take advantage of if they opt to educate themselves further on how to use hemp to better their overall health.

Despite the challenges of being classified as illegal because of the negative reputation of cannabis marijuana, CBD producing industrial hemp reemerged and carved its good reputation to the new world. It is showing its versatility and usability to combat health issues among humans and even their beloved canine companions.

It really pays to educate oneself on natural alternatives to the medication we usually take—all it takes is an open-mind, and the willingness to try new things. Who knows? This might be the very solution you've been looking for.

THANK YOU!

Before you go, I just wanted to say thank you for purchasing my book.

You could have picked from dozens of other books on the same topic but you took a chance and chose this one.

So, a HUGE thanks to you for getting this book and for reading all the way to the end.

Now I wanted to ask you for a small favor. **Could you please take just a few minutes to leave a review for this book on Amazon?**

This feedback will help us continue to write the type of books that will help you get the results you want. So if you enjoyed it, please let us know! (-:

59940299R00060

Made in the USA
Middletown, DE
23 December 2017